REVITALISE YOUR BODY

A comprehensive guide to conquering obesity, crushing cravings, shedding pounds and unleashing vibrant energy

By

Johnson N.Boyd

DISCLAIMER

A lady called Emily lived in the center of a busy

metropolis, where the smells of freshly made pastries and mouthwatering street cuisine mixed

together. She was vivacious, driven, and always on the move, managing her job, social life, and

family obligations with amazing grace. However, underneath her self-assured façade, Emily was

hiding a hidden battle that was silently eating away at her wellbeing and lurking in the

background of her busy existence.

Emily saw food as more than simply nourishment; it also represented joy, comfort, and

sometimes even sadness. Like many others, she discovered that when stress got to be too

much for her, she would go for munchies, finding solace in the comforting embrace of sweet or

salty delights. But as the years went by, Emily saw a pattern developing—a pattern of eating habitually rather than out of hunger.

One evening, as Emily sat in her little apartment, a wave of reflection passed over her. She

thought about all the hours she had wasted aimlessly snacking, the late-night refrigerator raids

motivated by boredom, and the grocery store impulsive purchases that often turned out to be

regrettable. That's when she saw she was caught in a vicious cycle—her eating decisions were

controlled by her hunger, which left her feeling helpless and unfulfilled.

Emily set out on a voyage of self-discovery, determined to take back control of her relationship

with food. This trip would eventually help her break free from the loop that was holding her

prisoner, comprehend the underlying causes of her eating patterns, and solve the riddles

surrounding hunger.

However, Emily's tale is not unique to her. Millions of people all across the globe may relate to this story—those who struggle with the complexity of contemporary eating habits, navigating a

world where convenience often takes precedence over nutrition and where emotional signals

can sometimes overwhelm physical hunger.

We explore the depths of this common conflict in "How to Break Free from the Hunger Habit,"

fusing scientific, psychological, and personal experience to reveal the secrets of our desire. We

investigate the processes behind our eating patterns and learn why we eat when we're not

hungry via engrossing narrative and perceptive analysis.

Each chapter reveals a new level of knowledge, enticing readers to set out on a life-changing

path of self-awareness and empowerment. Topics range from the complex dance between

biology and psychology to the potent effect of emotions and social dynamics.

We meet our own reflections in the mirror of Emily's problems as we travel with her and explore the depths of her experiences. We face the times when we are weak and vulnerable, the

temptations that seem to find us everywhere, and the mental battles we fight alone in silence.

However, hope endures despite the difficulties; it is a lighthouse that shows the way to

liberation. By means of awareness, introspection, and a strong will to transform, we learn that

overcoming the hunger habit is not only feasible but also a liberating journey that starts with one

little step and ends with a life full of satisfaction, vigor, and balance.

Thus, I cordially encourage you to accompany us on this incredible journey of self-discovery,

resiliency, and metamorphosis. Let's work together to solve the secrets behind the hunger habit,

take back control over food, and welcome a day when eating is a happy celebration of life rather

than just a basic human need.

TABLE OF CONTENTS

About the author

Johnson N. Boyd, the author of "Revitalize Your Body," is a seasoned health and wellness expert with over two decades of experience in the field. With a background in nutrition and fitness, Boyd brings a unique perspective to his writing, blending scientific research with practical advice. His passion for helping others achieve optimal health shines through in his work, making "Revitalize Your Body" a comprehensive guide for anyone looking to improve their physical well-being. Boyd's holistic approach emphasizes the importance of balanced nutrition, regular exercise, and mindfulness techniques for overall wellness. Through his clear and engaging writing style, he empowers readers to take charge of their health and transform their lives.

CHAPTER ONE

Comprehending the Habit of Hunger

First of all,

Investigating the underlying causes of hunger is essential

to deciphering the complexity of our eating behaviors. In

order to conduct this investigation, Chapter 1, "Revitalise your Body ," establishes the

foundation for comprehending the workings of our innate need to consume food.

The Origins of Hunger in Biology:

Fundamentally, hunger is a basic need for living. Our bodies have developed complex

mechanisms to detect hunger and control calorie intake, which have their roots in evolutionary

biology. The intricate web of hormones and neurotransmitters that affect our urge to eat is

orchestrated by the hypothalamus, a part of the brain that is critical for controlling hunger.

Leptin, often called the "satiety hormone," indicates fullness, whereas ghrelin, also called the

"hunger hormone," increases appetite.

But in addition to being controlled by physiological signals, hunger is also influenced by

psychological and environmental factors. The continual barrage of stimuli in today's food world

causes cravings and interferes with our body's normal hunger signals. It is essential to

comprehend these outside factors in order to successfully manage our eating habits.

The Mind of Hungry:

Beyond simple physiological demands, psychological variables have a profound impact on our

connection with food. Our eating habits are greatly influenced by a variety of factors, including

emotions, prior experiences, social standards, and cultural influences. For many people, eating

is a source of comfort, enjoyment, and social connection in addition to being a source of nourishment.

In addition, our brains are programmed to search for meals high in calories—a survival strategy

 refined over millions of years of evolution. When combined with contemporary food marketing

strategies, this natural predilection for high-calorie meals often results in overindulgence and

bad eating habits.

Ending the Cycle:

Knowing the hunger habit gives us the capacity to overcome harmful eating habits despite our

biological tendencies and external influences. Our eating habits may be reclaimed by practicing

mindfulness and awareness of our hunger signals. A better connection with eating may be

fostered by methods like mindful eating, which promote focusing on internal feelings and body

sensations related to food.

Making educated food choices also requires understanding the difference between physical

hunger and other forms of hunger, such as emotional or situational hunger. By understanding

the underlying causes of our desires, we may react to them in ways that support our long-term

health objectives.

Useful Techniques:

Offering doable tactics for maximizing the potential of comprehending the hunger habit, Chapter

1 ends here. These tactics include both more general social shifts and individual-level actions

targeted at encouraging healthy eating habits.

To overcome the hold of the hunger habit on an individual basis, mindful eating, food journals,

and self-compassion cultivation are useful techniques. Positive dietary habits may also be

maintained by cultivating a network of supporting people and surrounding oneself with

circumstances that encourage healthy eating.

At the social level, we may lessen the impact of outside influences on our eating patterns by

supporting laws that prioritize access to nutrient-dense foods, encourage food literacy, and

control food marketing to minors. By tackling the underlying reasons behind bad eating habits,

we may endeavor to establish a society that prioritizes health and nutrition.

In summary:

Chapter 1 clarifies the complex nature of hunger, laying the groundwork for a more in-depth

examination of human eating behaviors. We may actively cultivate healthy eating habits by

being aware of the biological, psychological, and environmental variables that influence our

connection with food. Equipped with understanding and consciousness, we may set out on a

path to recover mastery over our eating habits and nourish our bodies and minds for the best

possible health and wellbeing.

Why Do We Eat When We're Not Hungry? is the first chapter.

First of all,

In the contemporary world, food has many purposes than just sating hunger. We often eat when

we're not hungry because of a variety of reasons that go beyond simple physiological

requirements. "Beyond Hunger: Unveiling the Secrets of Our Eating Habits" explores the

psychological, social, and environmental factors that affect our eating habits in its first chapter,

which goes into great detail on the complexity of this phenomena.

The Emotional Psychology of Food

Our emotions, ideas, and prior experiences are intricately entwined with our connection with

food. When it comes to managing stress, worry, boredom, or other emotional states, food may

be a coping tool. When we turn to food for solace or diversion rather than actual hunger, this emotional eating often takes place.

Furthermore, our eating habits may be shaped by our upbringing and cultural background,

which can affect what, when, and how much we eat. Eating in social situations or consuming

certain meals out of habit or custom are examples of how social norms and expectations around

food may also have a big impact.

The Impact of the Food Environment

We are constantly being urged to eat by the current food environment, often even when we are

not hungry. Large portion sizes, food promotion, and easy availability to really appetizing meals

all lead to overindulgence and eating when not hungry. In addition, it's now simpler than ever to

engage in impulsive eating habits because to food availability and ease.

Moreover, food outlets are positioned and structured with the intention of encouraging consumption, creating an atmosphere that often encourages overindulgence in eating. Our

normal hunger signals may be suppressed by these environmental stimuli, which may result in

mindless eating and weight gain.

Biochemical Elements:

Biological reasons also contribute to the phenomena of non-hungry eating, even if psychological

and environmental variables are major contributors. Certain meals have the ability to take over

the brain's reward system, which is involved in controlling motivation and pleasure, resulting in

overeating and cravings.

Furthermore, dysregulation of leptin and ghrelin levels, among other hormonal abnormalities,

may interfere with our hunger signals and cause us to overeat even when we are not hungry. It

might be challenging to interrupt the vicious cycle of overeating and weight gain without help

due to these biological variables.

Ending the Cycle:

Breaking the pattern of non-hungry eating starts with understanding why we eat when we're not

hungry. We may start creating effective methods to address the emotional, social, and

environmental triggers that influence our eating patterns by identifying them.

We may better tune into our actual hunger signals and distinguish them from other forms of

hunger, including emotional or situational hunger, by engaging in mindfulness and

self-awareness practices. We may choose foods that are more mindful of our requirements by

learning to take a moment to think before we eat.

Reliance on food for comfort may also be decreased by learning other coping strategies for

handling feelings like stress or boredom. Emotional eating triggers may be managed by frequent

physical activity, relaxation exercises, or asking friends and family for assistance.

Useful Techniques:

Practical tactics for overcoming non-hungry eating are provided in the concluding section of

Chapter 1. These tactics center on helping people have a positive connection with food and

addressing the fundamental causes of our want to eat even when we're not hungry.

- Maintain a food journal. By recording what, when, and why you eat, you may see trends and

situations that lead to non-hungry eating. Making more thoughtful eating decisions may be aided

 by this understanding.

- Engage in mindful eating: Eating more slowly and carefully may make you eat less likely to

overeat by drawing your attention to the flavor, texture, and smell of the meal.

- Look for substitute coping strategies: Rather of reaching for food to soothe yourself, consider

 hobbies, exercise, or meditation as ways to better handle stress or emotions.

- Create a supportive environment: Assemble a team of individuals who share your commitment

to health and make changes to your house that will encourage healthy eating, such as

 minimizing the amount of time you spend with enticing foods and stocking your pantry with

 wholesome items.

In summary:

"Beyond Hunger: Unveiling the Secrets of Our Eating Habits" provides insight into the intricate

interactions among several elements that prompt us to eat even when we're not hungry in

Chapter 1. Through gaining knowledge of the psychological, social, and environmental factors

involved, we may take charge of our eating habits and have a more positive connection with

food. Equipped with information and techniques, we may more mindfully navigate the

 contemporary food landscape and make decisions that feed our bodies and brain.

CHAPTER TWO
The Science of Hunger

This chapter delves into the complex mechanisms behind hunger, examining its biological and

psychological aspects. Although hunger is a natural need that controls our eating habits, its

workings are far from straightforward. We will disentangle the complicated interactions that

occur between psychological signals, biological triggers, and the brain's complex control of

appetite and hunger.

1. Recognizing Biological Triggers

The body's intricate interactions between hormones, neurotransmitters, and brain circuits

govern hunger in the main. The hormone ghrelin, sometimes known as the "hunger hormone,"

is mostly generated by the stomach and stimulates appetite by acting on the brain's

hypothalamus. It is one of the main actors in the control of hunger. Ghrelin levels increase when emptying the stomach, alerting the brain to hunger. Nevertheless, ghrelin levels fall after eating,

which adds to satiety.

Another important hormone in the control of hunger is leptin, also generated by fat cells and

commonly referred to as the "satiety hormone." Leptin operates on the brain to suppress

appetite and manage energy balance. Leptin levels rise in situations when fat stores are

plentiful, informing the brain that energy reserves are adequate and reducing hunger. On the

other hand, appetite control may be upset in cases of leptin shortage or resistance, which may

result in overeating and obesity.

In addition to hormones, neurotransmitters like serotonin and dopamine are important in
controlling appetite and hunger. Eating triggers the release of dopamine, a neurotransmitter that

is often linked to reward and pleasure. Conversely, decreased serotonin levels have been associated with increased appetites for comfort foods and carbohydrates. Serotonin also plays a

role in mood regulation and hunger control.

2. Examining Psychological Set Points

Although biological variables play a crucial role in regulating hunger, psychological signals also

have a significant impact on our eating habits. Our connection with food is shaped by a variety

of elements, including emotions, acquired habits, cultural influences, and the environment.

Cues from the environment, such the sight and smell of food, may make people feel hungry and

make them eat more. Environmental factors such as food availability, promotion, and portion

sizes may also affect our eating habits, often resulting in overindulgence.

Our dietary habits, attitudes about eating, and food choices are shaped by cultural factors. Our

eating habits and food preferences are influenced by societal conventions, familial practices, and cultural traditions. For instance, overindulgence may be more prevalent in societies where

food is connected to festivities and get-togethers.

Hunger and eating habits are significantly influenced by emotions as well. Anxiety, boredom,

stress, and melancholy may all lead to emotional eating, a behavior in which eating is utilized as

a coping strategy for unpleasant feelings. Emotional eating often entails consuming comfort

foods that are rich in calories, which may result in bad dietary habits and weight gain.

Our eating habit is also influenced by learned behaviors that we acquire via experience and

training. For instance, we could be more inclined to seek out certain meals when we're feeling

anxious or depressed if we link them with comfort or pleasure. Likewise, if we develop the habit of using food as a reward or a form of discipline as children, these behaviors may carry over into

adulthood.

3. Uncovering the Brain's Function in Regulating Appetite and Hunger

The brain integrates information from the body, hormones, and environment to maintain energy

balance, which is crucial for controlling hunger and appetite. The main regulator of hunger and

satiety, the hypothalamus, is a little area near the base of the brain that plays a significant role in

this process.

The hypothalamus has many unique nuclei and circuits that regulate appetite and eating

patterns. Anorexigenic (appetite-suppressing) and orexigenic (appetite-stimulating) peptides, for

instance, are produced by neurons in the arcuate nucleus and operate on other areas of the

hypothalamus to control hunger and satiety.

Other brain areas, in addition to the hypothalamus, are involved in the control of appetite and

hunger. The mesolimbic pathway-based reward system, which involves dopamine and other neurotransmitters, is what drives food-seeking behavior and solidifies eating patterns. Food

preferences and portion sizes are influenced by the prefrontal cortex, which is also involved in

self-control and decision-making.

Furthermore, the gut-brain axis plays a key role in regulating appetite, according to new study.

The brain receives messages from the stomach via the vagus nerve, which carries nerve

impulses, and via the production of hormones such peptide YY and ghrelin. The gut's capacity

to communicate with the brain in both directions affects appetite and eating habits by providing

information to the brain about nutritional availability, gut motility, and satiety.

Developing tactics to encourage healthy eating and fight obesity requires an understanding of

the complex interactions between biological and psychological hunger cues. Researchers and healthcare providers may create more successful weight-management strategies and enhance

general health and well-being by focusing on the physiological as well as psychological aspects

of overeating.

..

CHAPTER THREE
Emotional Consumption

Emotional eating is a multifaceted phenomena whereby food is consumed in reaction to

emotional signals instead than actual hunger. This chapter examines the several emotional

factors that lead to overeating and talks about coping mechanisms for emotional hunger.

1. Identifying Emotional Stressors That Lead to Overeating

Many different feelings, such as stress, boredom, melancholy, loneliness, worry, and even

happiness, may lead to emotional eating. In times of emotional distress, food often acts as a

source of solace and diversion, offering some respite from unpleasant emotions.

One of the most frequent causes of emotional eating is stress. Stress causes our bodies to

produce chemicals like cortisol, which may enhance hunger and comfort food desires that are heavy in calories. Many individuals use food as a coping mechanism for stress, turning to sweet

snacks or decadent desserts to momentarily ease tension or worry.

Another strong emotional cause for overeating is boredom. We may resort to eating out of habit

or to find something enjoyable to occupy our time when we're bored. Emotional eating is often

linked to activities like mindless munching in front of the TV or grabbing for food out of pure

boredom.

Emotional eating may also be a result of sadness and loneliness, as individuals turn to food for

solace and company. Food may be a source of comfort during depressing or isolating moments,
offering momentary sensations of warmth and fulfillment.

An additional powerful inducer of emotional eating is anxiety. Individuals who are anxious could

use food as a coping strategy to calm their emotions and eliminate uncomfortable sensations, or

they might use it as a source of comfort or diversion.

Emotional eating may be triggered by even happy or celebratory feelings. Food is a major topic

of discussion at many social events and festivities, and individuals may overeat when they're

happy or excited.

2. Techniques for Handling Emotional Hungry

Although it might be difficult to quit the habit of emotional eating, there are a few techniques that

people can use to deal with their emotional hunger in a healthy way:

- Mindful Eating: Mindfulness training may make people more conscious of their eating patterns

and emotional cues. People may have more control over their eating habits and make more

deliberate decisions about what and when to eat by being aware of their emotions, hunger

signals, and the sensory experience of eating.

- Emotional Awareness: One of the most crucial initial steps in kicking emotional eating is recognizing and accepting your feelings. People may learn other coping mechanisms to meet

their emotional needs without resorting to food by increasing their awareness of the feelings that

lead to overeating.

- Healthy Coping Mechanisms: Breaking the pattern of emotional eating may be facilitated by

finding healthy coping mechanisms. Exercise, writing, meditation, and spending time with loved

ones are a few healthy ways to relieve stress and deal with boredom, worry, and grief.

- Building Resilience: People who are resilient and emotionally strong are better able to handle

life's obstacles without turning to food for solace. Developing healthy coping mechanisms,

creating social support systems, and engaging in self-care are all part of developing resilience.

- Nutrition Education: Acquiring knowledge about nutrition and how food affects mood and

energy levels might enable people to choose better foods and cut down on emotional eating.

People may discern between real hunger indicators and emotional demands by knowing the

difference between physical and emotional hunger.

Establishing a Supportive Environment: Resolving to stop emotional eating may be aided by

surrounding oneself with friends, family, or a therapist who can provide accountability and

encouragement. Establishing a support network may facilitate the adoption of constructive

coping mechanisms and the resolution of obstacles encountered along the journey.

- Seeking Professional Assistance: Consulting a therapist, counselor, or registered dietitian may

be helpful for those who are experiencing severe emotional eating disorders or underlying

psychiatric problems. These experts may provide tailored advice and assistance to address the

underlying reasons of emotional eating and create useful coping mechanisms.

People may break away from the cycle of emotional eating and develop a better connection with

food and their emotions by putting these ideas into practice and handling emotional hunger

proactively. Without resorting to food for solace, it is possible to cultivate better coping strategies

and nurture the body and spirit with patience and effort.

CHAPTER FOUR

Social factors affecting Eating Habits

We examine the significant importance of social factors on eating behavior in this chapter.

Our social environments greatly influence the foods we choose to eat and the habits we develop

when it comes to eating, stemming from cultural traditions, peer pressure, social standards, and

environmental signals. We'll examine the mechanics of peer pressure, how social norms affect

dietary decisions, and coping mechanisms for social pressure to overeat.

1. Social norms, Peer Pressure, and Dietary Decisions

The impact that peers or social groups have on a person's actions, attitudes, and choices is

known as peer pressure. Peer pressure may take many different forms when it comes to eating

behavior, ranging from overt encouragement or coercion to subliminal signals and standards

that mold our ideas of what constitutes appropriate eating behavior.

Adhering to social norms about food preferences and portion sizes is a prevalent kind of peer

pressure that has an impact on eating behaviors. At social events like get-togethers with family

and friends, or at meals with acquaintances, people may feel pressured, either consciously or

unconsciously, to imitate the eating habits of those around them.

Eating habits and food choices are also greatly influenced by social norms, which are the

unspoken guidelines and expectations that govern conduct within a community. These customs

may have a significant impact on anything from food choices and dietary restrictions to meal

scheduling and portion sizes, and they can differ greatly throughout countries, regions, and

social circles.

Adherence to social standards is further reinforced in many civilizations by the association of certain meals or eating patterns with rank, tradition, or social identity. For instance, denying food

may be seen as impolite or disrespectful in many cultures, yet sharing food with others is often

seen as a display of hospitality and charity.

Furthermore, as social media and digital platforms have grown in popularity, the impact of social

norms on eating habits has increased. Curated photos of food and dining events have shaped

ideas about what makes a "normal" or appealing meal.

2. Defying Social Pressure to Overindulge in Food

Even though societal effects on eating habits may have a significant impact, people can use the

following tactics to fight the urge to overeat and choose healthier options:

- Assertiveness: Refusing to give in to peer pressure and making autonomous eating decisions

may be facilitated by learning to speak up for one's own limits and preferences in social situations. People may maintain their commitment to their objectives and morals by politely

accepting food offers and voicing their dietary choices.

- Mindful Eating: During social meals, engaging in mindfulness practices may help people

become more aware of their feelings, hunger signals, and the social dynamics at work.

Regardless of societal pressures, people may make more thoughtful decisions about what and

how much to eat if they remain mindful of their own needs and remain in the present.

- Setting limits: People may steer clear of circumstances where they might feel under pressure

to overeat by setting clear limits with friends, family, and colleagues around food-related

activities. This might include recommending non-food-related social activities as an alternative

or imposing restrictions on the kinds of food that can be eaten in public.

- Building Supportive Networks: Refusing to give in to societal temptation to overeat may be strengthened and encouraged by surrounding oneself with friends, family, or neighbors who

share similar health objectives. Maintaining a healthy diet and navigating social settings may be

made simpler with the assistance of others.

- Planning Ahead: Making plans for social occasions or gatherings in advance might assist

people in identifying possible triggers for overeating and creating coping mechanisms for them.

This may include bringing a meal to share that fits with one's nutritional objectives, having a

nutritious snack before heading to an event, or placing a limit on decadent foods.

- Modifying the Environment: Modifying the physical or social surroundings may aid in lessening

the impact of societal influences on eating habits. This might include selecting eateries or

locations that provide better alternatives, promoting the use of healthier foods in public or professional contexts, or establishing social norms that put an emphasis on health and

wellbeing.

- Seeking Professional Support: Consulting a therapist, counselor, or registered dietitian may be

helpful for those who are dealing with enduring societal pressure to overeat or underlying

psychological problems connected to food and eating. These experts may provide individualized

advice and methods for combating societal impacts on eating habits.

People may adopt healthy eating habits and handle social circumstances with resilience and

confidence by putting these methods into practice and being proactive in handling social

pressures. Even in the face of societal norms and expectations, it is possible to resist peer

pressure and make decisions that are consistent with one's health objectives and beliefs with

experience and perseverance.

CHAPTER FIVE
Eating Consciously

We explore the notion of mindful eating in this chapter, which is based on mindfulness

meditation and stresses awareness, presence, and nonjudgmental attention to the eating

experience. In the end, mindful eating promotes people to develop a closer relationship with

their food, body, and senses, which leads to better eating practices and a more fulfilling

relationship with food. We will discuss the fundamentals of mindful eating, methods for

developing presence and awareness at the table, and approaches to delighting in food without

going overboard.

1. Developing Intention and Attendance at the Table

Cultivating awareness and presence at the table, paying attention to the sensory experience of eating, and being totally present in the moment are the first steps towards mindful eating. This is

observing ideas, feelings, and physical sensations that surface throughout the eating process in

addition to paying attention to the views, aromas, tastes, textures, and sounds of the meal.

Slowing down and appreciating each mouthful, taking the time to chew food properly and

completely enjoy its tastes and sensations, is one of the fundamentals of mindful eating. This

improves digestion and nutritional absorption in addition to making meals more enjoyable.

Paying attention to the body's natural signals of hunger and fullness rather than depending on

outside cues or emotional triggers is another component of mindful eating. People who eat

slowly and deliberately are better able to identify when they are really hungry and when they

have eaten enough, which helps them avoid overindulging and foster a positive connection with

food.

A non-judgmental attitude toward food and eating is another aspect of mindful eating. This

includes letting go of norms or previous conceptions about what is "good" or "bad" and

embracing each eating experience with acceptance, curiosity, and openness. When it comes to

choosing what to eat, this enables people to become more intuitive and trusting of their own

bodies.

2. Ways to Savor Food without Going Overboard

A person may avoid overindulging and enjoy eating thoughtfully by using the following methods

and practices:

- Mindful Meal Preparation: Mindful eating starts even before the food is placed on the table. A

more mindful eating experience may be facilitated by taking the time to plan and prepare meals

attentively, paying attention to ingredients, cooking techniques, and portion proportions.

- Setting the Scene: A welcoming, tranquil setting may improve the mindful eating experience.

This may include taking care while arranging the table, putting screens and other electronic

gadgets to the back of the room to reduce distraction, and pausing before meals to give thanks.

- Using All the Senses: During meals, using all the senses may improve and enrich the eating

experience. This involves enjoying the tastes on the tongue, smelling the aromas of food,

observing the textures as food is chewed and digested, and appreciating the colors and

presentation of food.

- Chewing Mindfully: By taking the time to chew food slowly and completely, one may improve

nutritional absorption and digestion as well as develop a greater awareness of the eating

process. Eating more slowly and mindfully may be achieved by counting the chews in each

meal or putting down utensils in between bites.

- Expressing Gratitude: Giving some thought to the food one eats may help one feel more

appreciative of and connected to the sustenance it offers. This might be thinking back on the

origins of the food or quietly appreciating the work that went into making the meal.

- Checking in with Hunger and Fullness: Throughout the meal, people may avoid overeating by

occasionally monitoring their hunger and fullness signals. This will help them determine when

they have had enough to eat. This entails stopping the meal in the middle to gauge one's level

of hunger or fullness and modifying portion amounts appropriately.

- enjoying Every mouthful: People should strive to completely experience the tastes, textures,

and feelings of food by enjoying each mouthful rather than speeding through meals. Chewing

gently, putting aside outside distractions, and allowing oneself to be totally present throughout

the eating experience are all part of this.

- Listening to the Body: People who have a greater understanding of their bodies' signals and

reactions to food are better able to make intuitive food choices and refrain from mindless

overeating. This entails being aware of emotional indicators that might affect eating behavior in

addition to bodily feelings like hunger, fullness, and contentment.

People may develop a more mindful eating style and increase their awareness, pleasure, and

enjoyment of food by adopting these methods and practices into their daily routine. In addition to

encouraging better eating practices, mindful eating feeds the body, mind, and spirit and

strengthens bonds between individuals and the environment.

CHAPTER SIX
Ending The Pattern

This chapter discusses methods for ending the vicious cycle of unhealthful eating patterns and

developing a good, balanced relationship with food. We will explore the skills and approaches

that may help people overcome their hunger habit and adopt a better lifestyle, from creating

good eating habits to useful advice for managing cravings and emotional eating.

1. Creating Nutritious Eating Practices

In order to break the cycle of harmful eating behaviors and to promote general well-being, it is

important to develop good eating habits. Eating healthfully entails providing the body with a

well-balanced, nutrient-dense diet while exercising restraint and attention while selecting foods.

The following are some essential guidelines for creating healthy eating habits:

Eat a Variety of Nutrient-Dense Foods: To make sure you're receiving a broad variety of vital

nutrients, try to incorporate a diversified selection of fruits, vegetables, whole grains, lean

meats, and healthy fats in your diet.

- Emphasis on Whole Foods: When compared to packaged and processed foods, whole,

minimally processed foods often have more nutrients and less added sugar, salt, and harmful

fats.

- Exercise Portion Control: Be mindful of dish sizes and steer clear of excessive portions,

particularly when eating out or snacking. To help you regulate quantities, use visual clues like

utilizing smaller dishes and bowls or comparing portion sizes to common items.

- Pay Attention to Your Body: Pay attention to the signals your body gives you about when

you're hungry and full, and eat when you need to. To savor every meal and appreciate the eating experience, practice mindful eating and refrain from eating out of boredom, stress, or

emotional triggers.

- Remain Hydrated: To promote general health and keep hydrated, sip plenty of water

throughout the day. Limit your intake of sugary drinks like soda and juice and replace them with

sparkling water, herbal tea, or water.

- Plan and Prepare Meals: To make sure you have wholesome alternatives on hand when

hunger hits, take the effort to plan and prepare meals in advance. Reducing dependence on

convenience foods and preventing impulsive food choices may be achieved by batch cooking,

meal planning, and stockpiling healthful snacks.

- Moderation, Not abstinence: When it comes to decadent meals or pleasures, use moderation

as opposed to severe abstinence. Give yourself permission to periodically indulge in your favorite foods, but watch how much and how often you eat them.

- Seek Balance: Include a range of foods from all food categories and savor a diversity of tastes,

textures, and cuisines to achieve a balanced diet. Steer clear of categorizing foods as "good" or

"bad" and strive for a generally balanced eating routine.

- Be Flexible: Recognize that dietary requirements and tastes may vary over time, and be

flexible and adaptive in your approach to eating. Accept flexibility and experimentation in your

diet; don't be scared to try new dishes or cooking techniques.

2. Realistic Advice for Kicking the Hunger Habit

It takes a mix of realistic tactics, mindfulness practices, and self-awareness to overcome the
hungry habit. The following useful advice will help you overcome typical obstacles and end the

vicious cycle of unhealthful eating habits:

- Recognize Triggers: Spend some time determining the factors, such as stress, boredom, emotions, or outside cues, that lead to harmful eating patterns. You may discover healthy coping

mechanisms and proactive methods to deal with these triggers by identifying them.

- Engage in Mindful Eating: During meals, cultivate mindfulness by focusing on the taste and

texture of food, observing your body's signals of hunger and fullness, and appreciating every

mouthful. A higher feeling of pleasure with food may be fostered and the cycle of mindless

eating broken with the aid of mindful eating.

- Keep a Food diary: Monitor your eating patterns by keeping a food diary that details what,

when, and why you consume. This might assist you in recognizing the emotional signals,

triggers, and patterns that can be causing overeating or other problematic eating behaviors.

- Stock Up on Nutrient-Dense, Healthful Options: Make sure your kitchen is always full with nutrient-dense, readily prepared, and palatable items. Making wholesome decisions and

avoiding the temptation of junk food or convenience meals may be made simpler by having

wholesome alternatives close at hand.

- Manage Your Stress: Learn healthy coping strategies to handle stress, such working out,

meditating, taking deep breaths, or going outside. You may lessen the chance of reaching for

food for consolation by managing your stress levels and figuring out better coping mechanisms.

- Seek Support: As you attempt to kick bad eating habits, surround yourself with encouraging

friends, family, or a medical professional who can provide accountability, direction, and support.

Maintaining focus and overcoming obstacles may be facilitated by having a support network in

place.

- Set Achievable and reasonable objectives: Rather than aiming for perfection, set attainable and reasonable objectives for yourself. Honor your progress with little triumphs and treat

yourself with kindness when you make mistakes or encounter obstacles. Recall that

perseverance and patience are necessary for transformation.

- Exercise Self-Compassion: Throughout the process of breaking the hungry habit, treat yourself

with kindness and compassion. Recognize that you are deserving of love and acceptance

regardless of your eating habits, and treat yourself with the same compassion and

understanding that you would provide to a friend.

- Remain Consistent: Despite obstacles or disappointments, never waver in your attempts to

adopt healthy eating practices. Make a commitment to altering your behavior for the better and

stay with it over time. Consistency is essential for creating new habits and ending old ones.

People may end the cycle of bad eating habits and develop a healthy, balanced relationship with food by putting these useful advice and techniques into practice. It is possible to overcome

cravings, emotional eating, and other barriers to long-lasting health and well-being with

mindfulness, self-awareness, and support.

CHAPTER SEVEN
The Environment's Function

This chapter examines the significant impact that our surroundings have on the foods we

choose to consume and the way we eat. The physical environment in which we eat, as well as

the social and cultural factors that impact our food perceptions, all contribute to the formation of

our eating habits and general health. We will explore methods for fostering a culture of healthy

eating and look at how different aspects of our environment influence the foods we choose to

consume.

1. Establishing a Friendly Environment for Nutritious Food

Developing settings, schedules, and social structures that encourage and support wholesome

food selections and constructive eating habits are all part of creating a welcoming atmosphere for healthy eating. Our physical surroundings, social networks, and cultural norms may all be

altered to facilitate the adoption and maintenance of healthy eating practices. The following are

some methods for setting up a setting that encourages eating healthily:

- Stock Up on Nutrient-Dense Foods: Make sure your house, place of employment, and other

often frequented places are well-stocked with a range of nutrient-dense, healthful foods. You are

more likely to pick whole grains, lean meats, fruits, veggies, and healthy fats when you have

ready access to them during times of hunger.

- Organize Your Kitchen: Set up your pantry and kitchen so that healthy options are easier to

find and more noticeable. Store unhealthy treats out of sight or in less accessible places, keep
fruits and veggies on the counter or at eye level in the refrigerator, and use transparent

containers to store meal prep materials and leftovers.

- Plan and Prepare Meals in Advance: To lessen dependency on convenience foods and

takeout, take the effort to plan and prepare meals in advance. Meal preparing, batch cooking,

and weekly menu planning may help you avoid impulsive eating by ensuring you always have

nutrient-dense alternatives on hand when hunger hits.

- Establish a Positive Eating Environment: A comfortable and laid-back dining space will help to

create the ideal atmosphere for satisfying and wholesome meals. Play relaxing music or have a

nice chat, set the mood with tablecloths, candles, or soft lighting, and practice mindful eating to

enjoy every mouthful of your meal and the whole dining experience.

- Reduce Food-Related Distractions: By shutting off electronics, refraining from multitasking,

and concentrating on the sensory aspects of eating, you may reduce distractions during meals.

You may avoid overeating and promote a higher feeling of pleasure with food by eating thoughtfully and paying attention to hunger and fullness indicators.

- Create Regular Eating Patterns: To give your eating plan structure and regularity, set regular

times for meals and snacks. A more balanced approach to eating is encouraged, excessive

hunger or grazing is avoided, and hunger and fullness signals are better regulated when meals

are taken at regular intervals throughout the day.

- Be in the Company of Supportive Peers: Assemble a support system of friends, family, or

coworkers who have similar health aspirations and beliefs. Supportive social networks may

provide motivation, responsibility, and useful assistance as you strive to maintain good eating

practices and overcome obstacles along the road.

- Set Healthy Boundaries: Specify expectations for food-related activities and social events with

friends, family, and/or colleagues. With confidence and firmness, state your dietary choices and objectives and politely refuse offers of unhealthy food or excessive indulgence.

- Engage in Self-Compassion: As you endeavor to establish a conducive atmosphere for a

healthy diet, treat yourself with kindness and compassion. Acknowledge that it takes time and

effort to make changes, and give yourself grace and leeway as you go through the ups and

downs of forming new routines and habits.

2. How Environment Affects Our Dietary Decisions

Our environment has a big impact on the foods we choose to consume and the manner we eat,

forming our habits, preferences, and perceptions in subtle but important ways. Numerous

elements of our surroundings, ranging from food accessibility and availability to social and

cultural eating customs, might influence the foods we choose to consume. The following are

some ways that our environment affects the foods we choose to eat:

Food Availability and Accessibility: Our eating habits and food choices are greatly influenced by

the availability and accessibility of food in our surroundings. Making wholesome decisions is

made simpler when there are healthy, reasonably priced alternatives available in grocery stores,

farmers' markets, and dining establishments; yet, food deserts and restricted access to fresh

produce may exacerbate unhealthy eating patterns.

- Environmental Cues and Triggers: The sight and scent of food, for example, might set off

appetites and affect dietary decisions. Fast food restaurants, vending machines, and food

commercials may all lure us to make snap decisions or bad decisions, particularly when we're

anxious or hungry.

- Social and Cultural Influences: Our eating habits and tastes are greatly influenced by social

and cultural conventions around food and eating. Social events, cultural practices, and family rituals all have a strong emphasis on food, which affects what, when, and how much we eat.

Our eating habits and food choices may also be influenced by peer pressure, societal

conventions, and the desire to blend in.

- Portion Sizes and Serving Procedures: These aspects of our surroundings might affect how

much we eat and lead to overindulgence. When meals is served family-style or in countries

where big portion sizes are customary, people may unknowingly take more calories than they

need. Similarly, using bigger bowls, plates, and utensils might cause people to overeat by

warping their perceptions of portion sizes.

- Marketing and Advertising: Food marketing and advertising have a significant impact on our

dietary preferences and choices by influencing our ideas of what foods are enticing, practical,

and accepted in society. The predominance of bad dietary habits and the intake of extra calories, sugar, and salt may be attributed to the advertising of unhealthy foods and drinks,

particularly to children and teenagers.

- Environmental Stressors and Triggers: Stressors related to the environment, such as financial

strains, traffic jams, or job deadlines, may affect how people eat by causing emotional eating,

comfort food cravings, or impulsive eating. Convenience and fast-food alternatives are readily

available in our surroundings, which might aggravate these inclinations and make it simpler to

make poor decisions while under pressure.

- Accessibility of Healthy alternatives: Our capacity to make nutrient-dense decisions and

sustain healthy eating habits might be impacted by the availability of healthy alternatives in our

surroundings. Poor dietary quality and health effects may result from communities' increased

reliance on processed and convenience meals due to a lack of fresh produce, grocery shops, and nutrient-dense food alternatives.

- Built Environment and Urban Design: Our communities' built environments and urban designs

have a variety of effects on the foods we choose to consume and the manner we eat. While the

availability of parks, food swamps, fast-food restaurants, and liquor shops might encourage bad

eating patterns and obesity, the existence of safe, walkable neighborhoods, parks, and

recreational facilities encourages physical exercise and healthy lives.

We may take proactive measures to foster a healthy eating environment and encourage good

eating habits and wellbeing by being aware of the ways in which our surroundings affect the

foods we choose to consume and the methods in which we eat. There are various ways to

construct settings that encourage healthy lifestyle choices and eating habits, from modifying our physical surrounds to cultivating social networks and cultural standards.

CHAPTER EIGHT
Handling Temptations and Cravings

This chapter delves into the subtleties of cravings and temptations, two potent forces that have

the ability to thwart even the most well-meaning attempts to eat healthfully. In order to achieve a

healthy and balanced relationship with food, we will explore the complexities of managing

cravings and temptations. This will include learning about the psychological and physiological

mechanisms underlying cravings as well as creating strategies for overcoming temptations and

choosing healthier options.

1. Recognizing Cravings and Managing Them

Strong cravings for certain meals or tastes are known as cravings, and they often have a

significant emotional or psychological component. Cravings are mostly caused by psychological, environmental, and social factors, while they may sometimes be brought on by physical hunger

or nutritional inadequacies. To successfully manage cravings and make better decisions, it is

important to comprehend the underlying reasons of desires. The following are some methods

for comprehending and controlling cravings:

- Recognize factors: Whether they be social, emotional, or environmental, spend some time

determining the factors that lead to your desires. Stress, boredom, emotions, food commercials,

social events, and exposure to enticing foods are common causes of cravings. You may lessen

the influence of these triggers on your eating decisions by identifying them and creating

proactive measures to deal with them.

- Develop Mindfulness: When you are needing something, practice mindfulness by focusing on

the here and now and paying attention to your feelings, ideas, and physical sensations. Without passing judgment or becoming attached, acknowledge the cravings as they occur and track

their ebbs and flows over time. Gaining more self-awareness and self-control via mindfulness

might help you react to cravings more expertly.

- Distract Yourself: When cravings hit, divert your attention from eating by doing chores or

activities that need both your body and mind. This may be taking a stroll, meditating or deep

breathing, reading a book, enjoying some music, taking up a hobby, or doing something

creative. You may ride out the wave of hunger until it passes by focusing your attention in other

directions.

- Attend to Underlying Needs: Cravings may sometimes be an indication that our bodies need

something else than food, such emotional support, stimulation, or comfort. Think about what

you're really needing for a minute, and see if there's anything else you can do to satisfy it than eating. For instance, you may look for a warm embrace or partake in a calming pastime that

makes you happy if you're in the need for comfort.

- Select Healthier Options: When cravings occur, seek for healthier options that will satiate your

needs while also supporting your wellness objectives. For instance, choose a tiny amount of

dark chocolate or a piece of fruit when you're desiring something sweet rather than sugary

snacks or desserts. Picking nutrient-dense foods that provide a harmony of taste, texture, and

pleasure can help you satiate cravings without going back on your diet.

- Exercise Moderation: Give yourself permission to periodically give in to your urges, but to

prevent overindulging, exercise moderation and portion control. Enjoy tiny portions of your

favorite meals attentively and relish every mouthful rather than going without entirely. You may

sate desires without jeopardizing your general health and wellbeing by include indulgences in your diet in a balanced and regulated way.

- Remain Hydrated: Especially if you're dehydrated, desires may sometimes be mistaken for

thirst signals. Drink lots of water, herbal tea, or other non-caloric liquids to stay hydrated

throughout the day. Try sipping a glass of water first when you have cravings to see if it helps

squelch your appetite.

- Get Enough Sleep: Sleep deprivation may interfere with hormones that control hunger and

cravings, increasing your susceptibility to unhealthy, high-calorie food desires. Make sure you

receive enough sleep every night to promote general health and wellbeing and lessen the

chance of cravings.

2. Techniques to Avoid Temptations and Make Healthier Decisions

Developing ways to resist temptations and make healthy choices when faced with food-related issues is just as important as controlling urges. Managing social events, avoiding food

promotions, and stifling the temptation to overindulge are just a few of the tactics that may

support you in staying on track and choosing better options. The following useful advice will help

you avoid temptation and make better decisions:

- Plan Ahead: Recognize when you're likely to succumb to temptation or make poor decisions,

and create plans in advance to lessen the effects of such circumstances. This may include

making a nutritious dinner before going to a social event, bringing a healthier dish to potlucks or

parties, or packing healthy snacks to take on the go.

- Set Boundaries: Clearly state your aims and preferences around eating, both to yourself and to

others. Don't be hesitant to politely and assertively express your limits, and don't be scared to

refuse meals or circumstances that don't support your health objectives. Establishing boundaries may assist you in maintaining focus on your objectives and fending off outside

pressure to make poor decisions.

- Practice Saying No: Develop the courage and conviction to say no to enticing foods or

circumstances. Remind yourself of the advantages of sticking to your objectives and the

reasons you are choosing to be healthy. Recall that declining unhealthy alternatives is not a sign

of deprivation but rather of self-care and respect.

- Use Visualizations: Envision yourself in difficult circumstances, making wise decisions and

stifling temptation. Imagine yourself navigating food-related issues with grace and

perseverance, feeling in control, powerful, and confident. You may reinforce beneficial actions

and fortify your commitment with the aid of visualizations.

- Seek Support: Assemble a network of friends, family, or neighbors that share your beliefs and aspirations for your health. When you try to avoid temptations and make better decisions, rely

on your support system for inspiration, accountability, and hands-on help. Maintaining focus and

overcoming obstacles may be made simpler with a solid support network.

- Exercise Self-Compassion: Show yourself kindness and compassion as you deal with

obstacles and disappointments connected to eating. Acknowledge that nobody is flawless and

that making mistakes from time to time is a common occurrence while trying to adopt better

habits. Practice self-compassion and treat yourself with the same consideration and

understanding that you would give to a friend, rather than concentrating on your faults or

condemning yourself.

- Keep an Eye on the Big Picture: As you negotiate food-related temptations and problems,

consider your long-term health and well-being. Instead of getting hung up on transient pleasures or disappointments, concentrate on the greater picture and the constructive adjustments you're

doing to improve your happiness and health. Keep in mind that every healthful decision

CHAPTER NINE
Physical Activity and Hunger

This chapter delves into the intricate connection between appetite and physical activity,

examining the ways in which exercise affects eating habits and feelings of hunger. We will look

at how physical activity affects our connection with food and our capacity to sustain good eating

habits, from the physiological processes that control appetite to the psychological effects of

exercise on hunger signals. We will also look at methods for controlling hunger and promoting

general wellbeing with exercise.

1. Investigating the Connection Between Exercise and Hunger

Numerous physiological, psychological, and behavioral variables interact to determine the

complex link between hunger and physical activity. Exercise may boost energy expenditure and produce a calorie deficit, which might reduce appetite temporarily in some people, but it can

also trigger hunger signals and cause them to eat more. Making educated decisions regarding

their exercise regimen and eating habits may be facilitated by having a thorough understanding

of the processes governing appetite and the impact of exercise on hunger.

- Physiological Mechanisms: A number of physiological processes play a role in how hunger

and appetite are controlled in response to physical activity. Changes in appetite and satiety

signals may result from physical activity's impact on hormone levels that control appetite,

including ghrelin, leptin, and peptide YY. Exercise may also improve food absorption and

stimulate hunger by increasing blood flow to the digestive tract.

- Psychological impacts: Exercise has important psychological impacts on appetite as well.

Mood, stress, and emotional state all have an impact on hunger signals and eating habits. Due

to variables like increased stress levels or mood swings, some people may find that after

exercising, their hunger increases, while others may find that their appetite decreases as a

consequence of physical activity's mood-enhancing benefits.

- Behavioral Patterns: The association between physical activity and hunger may also be

influenced by individual variations in eating habits, nutritional preferences, and exercise

routines. Following physical exertion, some people may indulge in compensatory eating habits,

ingesting more calories than they expended. Some people can have reduced appetites or see a

shift in their food choices that results in better eating practices.

2. How to Control Your Hunger and Encourage Healthy Eating with Exercise

Exercise may be a useful technique for controlling hunger and promoting good eating habits,

even if it can have complicated effects on appetite and eating behaviors. People may maximize

their exercise regimen to promote their general health and well-being by learning how to utilize

exercise strategically to control hunger and cravings. The following are some methods for use

exercise to control appetite and encourage a balanced diet:

- Timing of Exercise: Research suggests that exercising before meals may suppress appetite

and lower calorie consumption. Exercise timing may also have an influence on hunger signals

and appetite. It's important to experiment with various exercise schedules and see how they

effect your hunger and eating habits, since individual reactions to exercise scheduling may

differ.

Type and Intensity of Exercise: Certain types of exercise have a greater effect on the control of appetite than others. Exercise may also have an impact on hunger signals and appetite. While

moderate-intensity aerobic exercise may have less of an impact on hunger, high-intensity

interval training (HIIT) has been shown to reduce appetite in the short term.

- Balancing Energy Expenditure and Intake: Achieving a healthy balance between physical

activity and appetite management requires balancing the energy expenditure from exercise with

the energy intake from food. It's important to feed your body wholesome meals that provide you

the energy and nutrition you need to maintain your exercise regimen. You should also pay

attention to portion sizes and calorie intake to prevent consuming too many calories in excess of

what you burn off during exercise.

- Mindful Eating Practices: Including mindful eating techniques in your daily routine may help you improve your awareness of your body's signals of hunger and fullness and help you make

better decisions about what and when to eat. Take a minute to check in with your body and

gauge your degree of hunger before and after exercise. Then, eat thoughtfully to satiate your

hunger without going over or under.

Hydration: Maintaining proper hydration levels before to, during, and after physical activity is

crucial for promoting healthy hunger management and general wellbeing. Throughout the day,

particularly before and after physical activity, make sure to drink enough of water to avoid

dehydration, which may disguise hunger signals and increase sensations of hunger.

- Post-Workout Nutrition: Eating a well-balanced meal or snack after an exercise session that

consists of a mix of carbs, protein, and healthy fats will aid in muscle repair, energy storage

replenishment, and post-exercise recuperation. To maximize recuperation and sate hunger, try to have a nutrient-dense meal or snack 30 minutes to 2 hours after doing out.

- Consistency and variation: You may preserve appetite management and avoid boredom or

burnout by maintaining consistency in your exercise regimen and variation in the kinds of

activities you participate in. To keep things fresh and promote general health and wellbeing, combine a variety of aerobic, strength, flexibility, and balancing exercises into your regimen.

- Listening to Your Body: Using exercise to control appetite and promote good eating habits ultimately comes down to paying attention to your body's signals of hunger and fullness. Observe how various exercise modalities impact your hunger and eating patterns, then modify your exercise regimen and dietary choices to suit your needs.

Through the integration of these tactics into your daily exercise regimen, you may use the potential of physical activity to control your appetite, encourage wholesome eating practices, and attain enhanced general health. Keep in mind that each person will react differently to exercise and appetite management, so it's important to try out various strategies and pay attention to your body's signals to choose what suits you the best.

Exercise may be an invaluable ally in establishing and maintaining a positive relationship with food and fitness if it is done with awareness, balance, and consistency.

CHAPTER TEN
Durable Behaviours

In this last chapter, we emphasize the value of developing long-lasting habits for reaching and sustaining wellness and health objectives. Habits that can be sustained over time and result in long-lasting modifications to behavior and way of life are called sustainable habits. We will examine methods for forming enduring habits that enhance general well-being and encourage a balanced and meaningful life, from establishing realistic objectives to developing resilience and avoiding relapse.

- 1. Creating Reasonable Objectives for Prolonged Achievement

In order to create long-lasting habits, it is imperative that one sets realistic objectives. Achievable, quantifiable, and in line with your beliefs, objectives, and skills are realistic goals. You may steer clear of dissatisfaction and discouragement and gain momentum in the direction of long-term success by establishing realistic objectives. The following techniques may help you create reasonable objectives for sustained success:
- Determine Your Priorities: To start, decide what your wellness and health-related values and priorities are. Which elements of health and wellbeing are the most important to you? Establish priorities to guide your goal-setting process, whether it's increasing your level of

exercise, maintaining a healthy diet, controlling your stress, or getting enough sleep.

- Be Particular and Measurable: Establish precise, quantifiable objectives that give your efforts focus and direction. Instead of aiming for general objectives like "be healthier" or "lose weight," specify precise results that you can monitor and assess in real time. For instance, "exercise for 30 minutes five days a week" and "eat five servings of fruits and vegetables per day."

- Break Down Bigger objectives: To make bigger objectives more reachable and less intimidating, break them down into smaller, more doable tasks. Focus on achieving your objectives gradually by establishing modest benchmarks along the route, as opposed to attempting to make big changes all at once. As you reach each goal, acknowledge it and make use of it as inspiration to keep going.

- Establish Realistic Timelines: Based on your unique situation, obligations, and available resources, establish reasonable timelines for accomplishing your objectives. Setting high standards for yourself and pushing yourself are vital, but it's as critical to be realistic about the amount of time and work needed to reach them. As you work toward your objectives, be patient with yourself and adjust your deadlines as necessary.

- Put an Emphasis on Behavior Change: Give behavior change goals that emphasize creating enduring routines and habits priority over outcome-based objectives like weight reduction or fitness accomplishments. Establishing habits that promote long-term health and well-being may be achieved by concentrating on the process of behavior modification rather than simply the outcome.

- Track Your Progress: Regularly observe your activities, habits, and results to keep tabs on your progress toward your objectives. Track your exercise, food, sleep, and other health-related activities using tools like wearable technology, apps, and journals. Regularly assess your progress and, in light of your findings, modify your objectives or tactics.

- Seek Support and Accountability: As you work toward your objectives, surround yourself with encouraging friends, family, or a healthcare professional who can provide accountability, direction, and support. Talk to others about your objectives and ask them to assist you in staying motivated and on course. It might be simpler to overcome obstacles and maintain your commitment to your objectives when you have a support network in place.

- Celebrate Your Successes: No matter how little they may appear, acknowledge and appreciate your victories and accomplishments along the road. Take satisfaction in the measures you've done to reach your objectives and acknowledge your efforts and success. Honoring your achievements may provide you a greater feeling of self-worth, drive, and accomplishment, which will motivate you to keep pursuing your long-term objectives.

2. Sustaining Advancement and Avoiding Regression

Long-term maintenance of good behaviors depends critically on maintaining progress and avoiding relapse. Even while obstacles and failures are inevitable, there are techniques you may use to maintain your resilience and overcome difficulties. The following techniques may help you keep making progress and avoid relapsing:

- Remain Flexible and Adaptable: Recognize that life is full of unexpected turns and twists, and remain flexible and adaptable in your approach to behavior modification and goal-setting. If circumstances, priorities, or resources change, be ready to modify your expectations, plans, and objectives as necessary.

- Learn from Setbacks: Rather of seeing obstacles and setbacks as failures, see them as chances for development and education. When you have a setback, consider what went wrong, pinpoint possible causes or hindrances, and come up with plans on how to go over them in the future. Make the most of failures to hone your strategy and fortify your resolve.

- Exercise Self-Compassion: Show yourself kindness and compassion when you experience obstacles or failures on your journey. Give yourself the same consideration and compassion that you would give a friend, and acknowledge that obstacles are a typical part of the process of making long-term behavioral changes. To cultivate resilience and well-being, engage in self-care and self-compassion exercises.

- Put Progress, Not Perfection First: Embrace development and progress throughout time instead than focusing on perfection. Instead of setting impossible standards for yourself or hoping for faultless results, acknowledge and appreciate the strides you've taken and the constructive adjustments you've made to your life. Accept the path of constant progress and acknowledge that each step you take is a step in the correct way.

- Remain Connected to Your Why: Remain focused on the fundamental drives and rationale for your pursuit of your objectives, particularly under trying circumstances. Rekindle your feeling of purpose and dedication to your objectives by reestablishing your connection with your values, priorities, and ambitions. Remind yourself of the advantages reaching your objectives will bring to your life and general well-being.

- Manage Stress: Since stress may often serve as a trigger for relapse and harmful behaviors, it is important to develop good coping methods for handling stress and hardship. To encourage resilience and relaxation, include stress-reduction practices into your daily routine, such as yoga, deep breathing, mindfulness meditation, and spending time in nature.

- Celebrate Milestones and Achievements: To reinforce healthy habits and increase your drive and confidence, celebrate your triumphs along the road. Whether it's hitting a new health goal, following your diet for a week, or achieving a fitness milestone, take some time to recognize and enjoy your successes.

- Remain Consistent with good Routines: Remain constant with your routines and good habits even in the face of stress, hectic schedules, or interruptions. Even when life becomes busy, set aside time for stress relief, healthy food, exercise, and enough sleep as a priority. Long-term progress maintenance and relapse prevention depend heavily on consistency.

- Seek Support and Accountability: As you strive to sustain success and avoid relapse, rely on your support network for inspiration, direction, and accountability. Talk about your accomplishments, difficulties, and objectives with encouraging friends, family members, or a medical expert who can provide guidance, inspiration, and hands-on assistance. A solid support network helps keep you tenacious and dedicated to your objectives.

- Reflect and Reassess Frequently: Allocate time to consider your advancement, reevaluate your objectives, and modify your plans of action as necessary. You may learn from prior events and make well-informed judgments about your future objectives and activities by reflecting on your experiences, insights, and obstacles. Embrace experimentation, feedback, and ongoing development as you go through the ups and downs of changing your habit.

By using these techniques to your day-to-day activities,

CHAPTER ELEVEN
Wrap-Up

In this last chapter, we take stock of the path we've taken to overcome our hunger habit and develop a more positive, harmonious connection with food. In order to help us in our pursuit of better health and wellbeing, we've covered a broad variety of tactics and insights, from studying the physiology of hunger to managing cravings, working out, and developing long-lasting habits. We'll discuss the significance of accepting a new connection with food as we conclude our investigation and provide some closing comments on overcoming the hungry habit.

- Accepting a New Connection with Food

We have questioned popular beliefs about food and eating throughout this book, encouraging readers to reconsider their relationship with food and adopt a more deliberate and aware approach to nourishing themselves. A greater knowledge of the role that food plays in our lives, as well as the cultivation of mindfulness, compassion, and respect for our bodies and ourselves, are all part of embracing a new relationship with food. The following are some essential ideas to keep in mind when we work to develop a better connection with food:

1. The practice of mindful eating involves paying attention to hunger and satiety indicators, appreciating each meal, and practicing mindfulness and presence throughout the eating process. We may improve our enjoyment of food, increase our sense of fullness, and make more deliberate decisions about what and how much we eat by taking our time and focusing on the sensory aspects of eating.

2. Rather than depending on outside guidelines or limitations, intuitive eating promotes trusting our bodies' natural signals of hunger, fullness, and contentment. We may cultivate a more harmonious connection with food and advance general well-being by learning to listen to our bodies' natural signals and acknowledging our hunger and urges without passing judgment.

3. feeding Over Nutrition: Rather than concentrating simply on the nutritional value of food, we should also consider the emotional, social, and cultural components of eating as well as the physical aspects of feeding. We may develop a more holistic approach to eating that promotes our general health and vitality by giving priority to foods that feed our bodies, brains, and spirits.

4. *Food as Fuel and Pleasure: Seeing food as both fuel and pleasure enables us to maintain a healthy balance between treating ourselves to the odd treat or indulgence and providing our bodies with nutrient-dense meals. We may have a more fulfilling and pleasurable connection with food that fosters contentment and

wellbeing by embracing our appetites and indulging in food without feeling guilty or constrained.

5. Self-Compassion and Self-Care: Developing a healthy connection with food and our bodies requires engaging in self-compassion and self-care practices. We may overcome self-destructive habits of guilt, shame, and self-criticism and develop a stronger sense of self-worth and wellbeing by being kind, understanding, and accepting of ourselves.

Concluding Remarks on Eliminating the Hunger Habit

As our quest to overcome the hungry habit draws to an end, it's critical to take stock of our accomplishments and the knowledge we've gained. Gaining control over the hunger habit is a continuous process of self-awareness, development, and change rather than a single event. Here are a few closing ideas to keep in mind as we go on our journey to improved health and wellbeing:

1. Accept Imperfection: Recall that overcoming the hunger habit is more about making progress and picking up lessons from our mistakes than it is about reaching perfection. Recognize that obstacles and disappointments are a normal part of the transformation process and treat yourself with kindness as you embrace the adventure.

2. Trust Yourself: When navigating the complexity of food and eating, trust your gut feelings, inner guidance, and intuition. Honor your urges, pay attention to your body's cues, and have faith in your ability to make wise decisions that promote your health and wellbeing.

3. Develop Resilience: Develop tenacity and resilience in the face of challenges and disappointments. It takes perseverance, resolve, and resilience to overcome obstacles and remain dedicated to your objectives in order to create enduring habits and conquer the hungry habit.

4. Celebrate Your Progress: Regardless of how little or unimportant it may seem, acknowledge and appreciate your accomplishments. On your path to improved health and wellbeing, every stride you take, every good decision you make, and every instance of self-awareness is a win worth acknowledging and applauding.

5. Keep Your Support System Connected: When you need direction, inspiration, or accountability, reach out to friends, family, or a medical professional. Embrace the company of like-minded individuals who will encourage and support you along the way and provide insight and direction when you most need it.

6. Be Open to development: As you go on your journey toward improved health and wellbeing, have an open mind to new opportunities, development, and change.

Accept chances to learn, explore, and find more about yourself. You should also be open to stepping outside of your comfort zone to try new things and break bad habits.

In summary, overcoming the hunger habit is a path of self-awareness, development, and change that calls for endurance, self-compassion, and patience. We may design a balanced, satisfying, and meaningful existence by adopting a new relationship with food, developing sustainable habits, and remaining dedicated to our health and well-being. May we emphasize self-care, self-compassion, and self-love as we go on our path, understanding that our wellbeing is worth the time and work it demands.

CHAPTER TWELVE
Resources for Ongoing Development and Education

It is crucial to continue learning and developing in order to break the cycle of hunger and promote a better connection with food and nutrition. In order to help people in their ongoing quest of knowledge and growth in the fields of nutrition, health, and personal development, Chapter 12 of the book "Hunger Habit" provides suggestions for further reading, resources, and support networks. In the quest for optimum health and well-being, this chapter recognizes that while the other chapters have offered a basis for understanding and managing the hunger habit, there is always more to learn and explore.

Additional Reading:

1.   Books on Health and Nutrition:
- Michael Pollan's book The Omnivore's Dilemma* examines how contemporary food production affects society, the environment, and health.
- Michael Pollan's In Defense of Food: An Eater's Manifesto*: Offers advice on choosing better foods and comprehends the significance of nutrition for general wellbeing.
- Michael Pollan's Food Rules: An Eater's Manual* provides easy-to-follow instructions for eating sensibly and healthily.

- Dan Buettner's book The Blue Zones: Lessons for Living Longer From the People Who've Lived the Longest explores the eating and lifestyle patterns of those who live in areas where life expectancy is very high.
- Evelyn Tribole and Elyse Resch's Intuitive Eating: A Revolutionary Program That Works: Promotes a non-diet approach to eating that is centered on paying attention to and respecting the body's signals of hunger and fullness.

2. Articles and Journals on Nutrition and Health:
- Nutrition Today: A peer-reviewed publication that discusses public health, nutrition research, and dietary recommendations.
- The Nutrition Source (Harvard T.H. Chan School of Public Health): Offers materials and articles on nutrition and healthy eating that are supported by research.
- American Journal of Clinical Nutrition: disseminates findings on dietary therapies, clinical nutrition, and the connection between dietary habits and health consequences.

3. Meditation and the Psychology of Eating:
- Jean Kristeller and Alisa Bowman's The Joy of Half a Cookie: Using Mindfulness to Lose Weight and End the Struggle with Food* offers mindfulness practices for controlling cravings and encouraging better eating practices.
- Savor: Mindful Eating, Mindful Life by Lilian Cheung and Thich Nhat Hanh: This book examines the

connections between eating and mindfulness and provides strategies for developing a more mindful relationship with food.

Instruments:

1. Apps for Meal Planning and Tracking:
- MyFitnessPal: A well-known app to monitor activity, food consumption, and dietary objectives.
- Let Go!Assists users in creating individualized dietary and weight reduction goals and monitoring their advancements over time.
- Mealime: Provides individualized recipes and meal plans based on dietary requirements and wellness objectives.

2. Health and Nutrition Trackers:
- Cronometer: Monitors consumption of micronutrients and offers a thorough nutritional analysis of meals.
- Fooducate: Reads food labels and offers insights into product components as well as nutritional data.
- NutrientIQ: Evaluates eating patterns and offers tailored suggestions to enhance nutrient intake.

3. Cooking and Recipe List:
- Allrecipes: An extensive library of recipes, culinary advice, and meal ideas contributed by users.
- preparation Light: Provides wholesome meal ideas, preparation methods, and nutritional guidance.
- Minimalist Baker: Focuses on simple, plant-based dishes with less preparation time and supplies needed.

Encouragement of Further Growth:

1. Online forums and communities:
- r/nutrition (Reddit): A discussion board for dietary plans, nutrition science, and healthful eating practices.
- MyFitnessPal Community: An online community where members may ask for help, relate success stories, and trade diet and exercise advice.
- Healthline Nutrition Community: A forum for exchanging stories, asking queries, and getting access to research-backed dietary advice.

2. Nutritional Guidance and Coaching:
- Precision Nutrition: Provides tools and individualized nutrition coaching programs to help people reach their fitness and health objectives.
- Registered Dietitian Nutritionists (RDNs): Certified experts offering individualized assistance and guidance in nutrition.
- Practitioners of Health at Every Size (HAES): Prioritize the promotion of holistic health and wellbeing, irrespective of weight or body type.

3. Programs for Wellness and Fitness:
- Peloton Digital: Offers anywhere-accessible on-demand fitness sessions, such as weight training, yoga, and meditation.
- ClassPass: Provides access to a range of studios and fitness classes, enabling customers to experiment with various exercises and training regimens.

A well-known YouTube channel that offers free yoga courses to practitioners of all skill levels is called Yoga with Adriene.

IN SUMMARY

People may keep moving forward in their quest to break the habit of hunger and develop a better connection with food and nutrition by making use of the tools and networks of support that are described in Chapter 12. The secret is to stay dedicated to continuous learning and improvement in pursuit of optimum health and well-being, whether via more reading, the use of tools and applications, or seeking assistance from online groups and specialists. People may empower themselves to make educated decisions, build enduring habits, and succeed in their quest for a better lifestyle with commitment and efforts.

www.ingramcontent.com/pod-product-compliance
Lightning Source LLC
Chambersburg PA
CBHW051828250726
48659CB00005B/1730